Ana Claudia M. Rangel de Abreu

Endometritis in dairy cows

Ana Claudia M. Rangel de Abreu

Endometritis in dairy cows

Causes, diagnosis, prognosis and treatment

ScienciaScripts

Cover image: www.ingimage.com

This book is a translation from the original published under ISBN 978-3-330-99889-6.

Publisher:
Sciencia Scripts
is a trademark of
Dodo Books Indian Ocean Ltd. and OmniScriptum S.R.L publishing group

120 High Road, East Finchley, London, N2 9ED, United Kingdom
Str. Armeneasca 28/1, office 1, Chisinau MD-2012, Republic of Moldova, Europe
Printed at: see last page
ISBN: 978-620-8-20560-7

Index:

LITERATURE REVIEW ENDOMETRITIS IN DAIRY COWS

SUMMARY

The economic viability of dairy herds is closely linked to the reproduction of these animals. Endometritis, also known as genital catarrh, is an inflammatory process involving only the endometrium and is responsible for major economic losses due to the reproductive failure it causes. There are some risk factors that contribute to increasing the incidence of endometritis in cows, such as retained placenta, poor hygiene at the calving site, dystocia, twin births and nutritional disorders. Therefore, knowing the predisposing factors for the occurrence of endometritis, it is possible to establish forms of prevention, involving the management and nutrition of cows during the transition period. Gynecological examination of cows during the puerperium period is recommended in order to diagnose and treat uterine infection early. Currently, there is a wide range of drugs that can be used to treat endometritis, but due to the shortage of milk, prevention remains the most cost-effective measure for producers.

1. INTRODUCTION

Reproduction is one of the main pillars of milk production (LEBLANC, 2008). The goal of dairy cattle reproduction management is to get cows pregnant efficiently and with a profitable calving interval. Although there are many causes of poor reproductive performance in lactating cows, veterinary medicine has focused on the pre- and post-partum management of these animals (LEBLANC et al., 2002).

Uterine diseases are known to cause economic losses due to a drop in milk production, lower pregnancy rates, an increase in the service period, an increase in the calving interval and an increase in the culling of cows due to reproductive failure (LEBLANC et al., 2002; SHELDON et al., 2009). The period leading up to calving, as well as the first few weeks after calving, the so-called transition period, are very important for the success of a new dairy cow pregnancy (KOZICKI, 1998).

For this reason, it is important to know the risk factors for uterine diseases in the puerperium and reduce their effects on the reproductive performance of dairy cows.

2. PUERPERIUM IN COWS

The postpartum period, also known as the puerperium, begins with the birth of the product until the period in which the maternal organism recovers from the transformations resulting from gestation, allowing the female to be fit for a new pregnancy (HAFEZ, 2004). At the time of delivery and during the first few days of puerperium, the uterus is heavily contaminated by microorganisms present in the environment. In the first week of puerperium there is a mixed uterine infection, in which a wide variety of microorganisms are present, but mainly coliforms. In the third and fourth weeks after delivery, this bacterial population decreases and is replaced by *Corynebacterium pyogenes* bacteria, which establish synergism with gram-negative anaerobic bacteria of the *Fusobacterium spp.* and *Bacterioides spp.* genera (GRUNERT et al., 2005). If the organism is unable to eliminate this bacterial contamination, uterine disease sets in.

The puerperium can be divided into two phases: the first, called delivrment, corresponds to the release of the fetal secondaries which should occur between six and twelve hours after delivery and the second phase corresponds to macro and microscopic uterine involution and preparation of the uterus for a new pregnancy (PRESTES & ALVARENGA, 2006). During these phases, the endometrium regenerates, ascending bacterial contamination is eliminated and normal ovarian activity resumes. Therefore, a cow's lifespan is directly related to the events that take place during the puerperium. The rapid return to reproduction allows for a new conception up to 90 days after calving, enabling a calving interval of 12 months (KASK et al., 2003).

The contractions of the myometrial muscle fibers are responsible for eliminating bacterial agents and promoting the restoration of the uterus to its normal morphology and endometrial regeneration (HAFEZ, 2004). Normal postpartum uterine discharges are composed of the remains of fetal membranes and fluids, maternal tissues, blood and mucus, and due to their composition they constitute an environment conducive to the development of bacteria. The appearance and smell of these discharges are important clues to the presence and/or severity of uterine diseases. Discharge from the loops usually begins on the 3rd day postpartum and continues until the 10th day (REBHUN et al., 2000), and during this period the appearance of the loops changes from a brownish-red liquid to a yellowish-white, viscous material (SHELDON et al., 2006). However, if there is a delay in uterine involution, loach elimination can continue up to 4 weeks postpartum (DROST et al., 2002).

For the endometrial epithelium to recover, there must be vasoconstriction in the caruncles, causing vascular degeneration and peripheral ischemia, and consequently the detachment of necrotic tissue from the uterine wall (SENGER, 2003).

Uterine and cervix involution ranges from 25 to 47 days (MORROW et al., 1966; HARRISON et al., 1986). However, involution of the cervix is slower than that of the uterine body and horns due to the large amount of collagen that makes up its cervical rings (MORTIMER et al., 1997). Complete microscopic uterine involution takes longer than palpable macroscopic involution, ranging from 42 to 50 days (MARION & GIER, 1959). The table below shows the characteristics that can be assessed by rectal palpation during the gynecological examination in the puerperium.

Uterine involution	Characteristics on rectal palpation
1	Uterus completely in the abdominal cavity.

2	Only the beginning of the uterine horns can be palpated.
3	Palpation of more than half of the uterus in the abdominal cavity.
4	Access to the entire uterus, but still in the abdominal cavity.
5	More than half of the uterus in the pelvis.

Table 1: Macroscopic characteristics related to uterine involution assessed by rectal palpation during the puerperium of cows. **Source:** (FERNANDES & FIQUEIREDO, 2007).

It is possible to speed up the process of uterine involution and thus reduce the incidence of uterine infections with the use of PGF2a analogues in postpartum dairy cows, as it acts to expel the lochia and contaminated contents due to its uterotonic effect (FERNANDES & FIGUEIREDO, 2007). The earlier the estrus of the animals in the puerperium, the faster the uterine involution will occur, and under the influence of estrogen, the immune defense of the uterus is enhanced, in addition to favoring the production of mucus and helping to clean the uterine lumen (HORTA, 1995).

There are a number of factors that directly affect the process of uterine involution in cows, including: number of calvings, age, concomitant puerperal disorders, shaving and return of ovarian activity. In relation to the number of calvings, primiparous cows show faster uterine regression than multiparous cows (KOZICKI et al., 1984; ZAIN et al., 1995). In an experiment carried out by GONZALEZ SANCHEZ et al. (2008), it was found that the uterus of cows with a greater number of calvings remains in the abdominal cavity for a longer period of time, contributing to the importance of the uterus' positioning during the process of eliminating the loops in the puerperal phase. Fibrosis, relaxation of the muscle cells and of the supporting ligaments are physiological alterations that occur in the uterus of older animals with a greater number of births, leading to a decrease in the contractility of the uterus during the involution process (GONZALEZ SANCHEZ et al., 2008). Similarly, the uterus of cows with calving complications involutes more slowly than that of cows with eutocic calving (SHELDON, 2007). According to NOGUEIRA et al. (1993), *Bos taurus taurus* animals have slower uterine involution than *Bos taurus indicus* animals *and* are therefore less predisposed to the occurrence of postpartum uterine diseases.

With regard to the return of cyclicity postpartum, it is known that uterine disease can negatively influence ovarian activity. In addition, endotoxins resulting from gram-negative bacteria decrease the sensitivity of the anterior pituitary gland to GnRH, inhibiting the pulsatile release of LH (HARRIS et al., 2000; WILLIAMS et al., 2001), which is responsible for follicle growth and ovulation. However, in cows with normal puerperium, the onset of ovarian activity usually occurs between 15 and 30 days of the postpartum period (GRUNERT et al., 2005), with the first postpartum estrus without behavioral signs occurring around the 15th day, the second between the 32nd and 33rd days, and the subsequent ones in regular 21-day cycles (REBHUN et al., 2000).

3. UTERINE IMMUNITY

The immune function of the uterus is decreased in dairy cows from one to two weeks before calving to two to three weeks after calving (MALLARD et al., 1998). This is due to a negative energy balance, mobilization of body fat and protein, changes in oestrogen and progesterone levels at the end of gestation and an increase in cortisol levels during calving (STRATEN et al., 2008 and GALVAO et al., 2009).

The control of uterine infections is related to the activation of organ defenses, consisting of mechanical, immunological and hormonal factors (Table 2). Thus, under physiological conditions, the uterus is capable of efficiently eliminating bacterial infection.

1. Mechanical factors:	- Closing of the vulva - Cervix - Uterine motility - Uterine secretion
2. Immunological factors:	- Neutrophil migration - Phagocytic cells (neutrophils and macrophages) - Specific opsonins - Immunoglobulins (IgG. IgM, IgA)
3. Hormonal factors:	- Estrogen - Progesterone
	- Prostaglandin
4. Stages of the estrous cycle:	- Follicular phase - Lutein phase

Table 2: Uterine defense mechanisms.

The innate or non-specific defense mechanisms of the female reproductive tract are made up of anatomical barriers (vulva and cartilaginous rings of the cervix) and physiological barriers (cervical mucus which prevents bacterial contamination) and the action of polymorphonuclear cells (neutrophils and macrophages) against microorganisms (SHELDON & DOBSON, 2004). As childbirth approaches, the anatomical barriers become dilated, facilitating the penetration of microorganisms (CAMARGOS et al., 2013). And neutrophils and macrophages are mobilized into the uterus resulting in transient leukopenia followed by neutrophil left shift (DETILLEUX et al., 1995).

In addition to innate immunity, there is also an acquired immune response made up of humoral and cellular immunity. Humoral immunity in the form of immunoglobulins is responsible for the opsonization of bacteria so that they can be phagocytosed by polymorphonuclear cells and the activation of the complement system (SINGH et al., 2008). In the presence of uterine infection, WATSON et al, (1990) found an increase in immunoglobulin titers in the uterus and vagina, but no change in serum levels. IgA, found in vaginal mucus, is the main immunoglobulin that protects against pathogens in the caudal portion of the reproductive tract, while IgG protects the uterus against bacteria and toxins.

Bacterial antigens captured by antigen-presenting cells stimulate T Helper lymphocytes to produce interleukin-2, which stimulates B lymphocytes to produce specific antibodies to fight infection (SINGH et al., 2008).

The interaction of these mechanical and immunological factors with the phases of the estrous cycle must be considered, since ovarian activity has a direct effect on the uterus in terms of resistance to and elimination of bacterial infections. Estrogenic influences on the uterus prevent infection, while prolonged levels of progesterone make the uterus more susceptible. Estrogen is responsible for stimulating epithelialization, vascularization of the endometrium, increased production of cervical mucus and secretions from the oviduct, uterine contraction, and sexual receptivity (BONDURANT, 1999), but mainly for enhancing neutrophil function (REBHUN et al., 2000). In contrast to the action of oestrogen, progesterone acts against uterine contractility, promotes the differentiation of endometrial glands and a reduction in the amount of cervical mucus, as well as having an immunosuppressive effect (BONDURANT, 1999). Therefore, in cows with a functional corpus luteum, exogenous administration of PGF2a is used to stimulate luteolysis, reduce progesterone and increase estrogen concentrations by inducing estrus with the aim of resolving endometritis (SHELDON et al., 2006).

4. PREDISPOSING FACTORS

Uterine infections can be classified as specific, when they develop without predisposing causes and are characterized by their enzootic nature (campylobacteriosis, brucellosis) or unspecific, when they require a predisposing cause and affect individual animals in the herd. Endometritis can occur during the puerperal and post-puerperal periods and after copulation or insemination when contaminated bulls or semen are used. With regard to puerperal endometritis, more than 90% of cows have uterine bacterial contamination in the first 15 days postpartum, declining to less than 20% in the 60 days postpartum, due to the defense mechanisms of the uterus. However, when defenses are deficient, these bacteria can grow and colonize the uterine environment, leading to disease. And post-puerperal endometritis is favored when there is functional insufficiency of the cervix due to functional disorders of the ovaries and insufficient closure of the vulvar lips (CAMPOS & CARRER, 2007).

The table below summarizes the main factors that can predispose cows to endometritis.

1. Anatomical and mechanical factors:	- insufficient closure of the vulvar lips - impaired occlusion of the cervical canal - impaired uterine contractility making it difficult to eliminate uterine contents

2. Pregnancy and childbirth disorders:	- miscarriages of infectious or sporadic origin - twin pregnancy - fetal death (mummification/fetal maceration) - dystocia - caesarean section/ fetotomy - childbirth indulgence - retention of fetal membranes
3. Uterine changes during pregnancy:	- uterine atony - uterine torsion - closure of the cervix before elimination of the secundins
4. Poor reproductive management:	- failure to control herd health - management deficiency at the end of the
	pregnancy, childbirth and puerperium - lack of hygiene during childbirth - tragao forgada do bezerros - placental abruption - failure to treat retained placenta
5. Organic deficiencies:	- ketosis, hypocalcemia - estrogen and progesterone
6. Nutritional management:	- low ECC - fat cows at calving
7. Associated illnesses:	- brucellosis, IBR-BVD, leptospirosis, salmonellosis, trichomonosis

Table 3: Predisposing factors for the occurrence of puerperal and post-puerperal endometritis in dairy cows.

There is a strong relationship between retained placenta and puerperal endometritis, with approximately 25-50% of cows with retained placenta developing endometritis (LEBLANC, 2008). This relationship is often associated with abortion, dystocia, multiple births, longer gestation, induction of labor, fetal anasarca, fetotomy and uterine prolapse (REHBUN, 2000). Another factor to consider is the fact that there is an immune deficiency associated with placental retention before and after calving, contributing to cases of endometritis in these cows (HORTA, 1995).

In cows, endometritis is also associated with inadequate vulvar angulation and calving problems (MARKUSFELD, 1987; CORREA et al., 1993; KIM & KANG, 2003; HAN & KIM, 2005; POTTER et al., 2010). Because during dystocia, tissue damage often occurs, causing devitalization, and obstetric interventions contribute to an increase in the pathogen load in the uterus. Other risk factors for endometritis are dirty facilities during delivery, uterine atony and iatrogenic vaginal contamination (REBHUN et al., 2000).

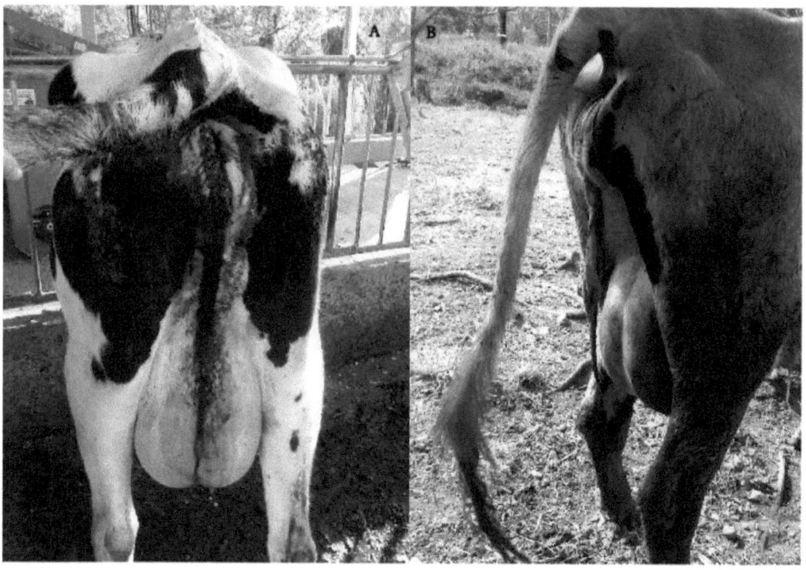

Figure 1: Predisposing factors for endometritis: A, Vulva laceration in a

Holstein cow due to dystocia; B, Retained placenta in a Holstein cow treated for hypocalcemia. **Source:** Personal archive.

Some studies have shown an association between age and the incidence of uterine infection (BRUUN et al., 2002), with SMITH & RISCO (2002) stating that the lowest incidence occurs in cows between 2 and 4 years of age and the highest incidence in cows over 7 years of age due to the increase in postpartum problems. However, LEWIS (1997) found the opposite, that cows between 2 and 4 years of age are more prone to dystocia and retained placenta and therefore have a higher incidence of uterine infections.

The time of year when calving takes place can also influence the incidence of endometritis. The hottest months of the year are associated with an increase in reproductive abnormalities due to the effect of heat stress on the cow's metabolism and immunity (QUINTELA et al., 2004).

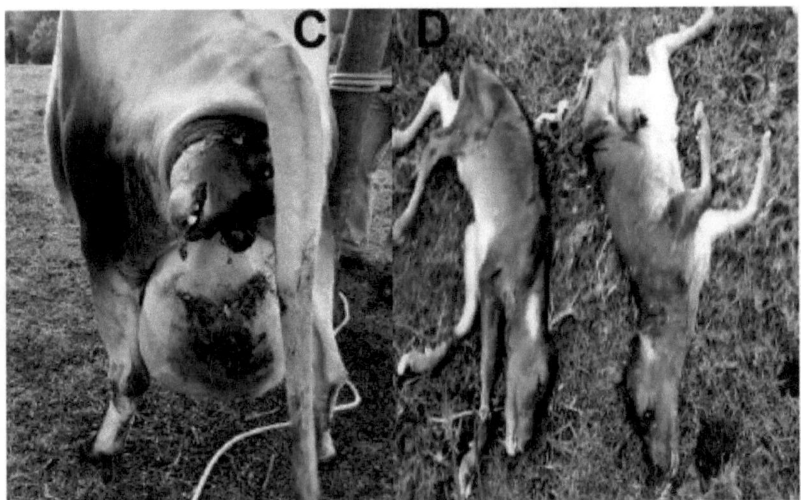

Figure 2: Predisposing factors for endometritis: C, Dystocia in a Jersey cow; D, Twin birth. **Source:** Personal archive.

In relation to nutritional management, a low body condition score during the drying off period and a high body condition score at the time of calving are related to a greater risk of dystocia and retained placenta and, consequently, endometritis (VASCONCELOS et al., 2000). Poor nutrition can lead to uterine infections by weakening the animal's immune system (LEBLANC et al., 2011; MARTINS, 2010), and a negative energy balance (NEB) increases the chances of uterine infections developing (KONYVES et al., 2009).

Metabolic disorders such as hypocalcemia and ketosis can also predispose cows to endometritis. REIST et al. (2003) state that cows with concentrations of more than 0.4mmol of acetone per liter of milk are at greater risk of developing uterine disease. Suggesting that this could be a way of identifying these animals and promoting appropriate interventions.

5. ETIOLOGY OF ENDOMETRITIS

The etiology of endometritis is multifactorial, with a wide variety of etiologic agents (Table 4) and predisposing factors. However, the majority of endometritis in dairy cows is bacterial in origin (FOLDI et al., 2006). Bacterial contamination of the uterus at the time of calving comes from the environment, the skin and the cow's own feces. Thus, *E. coli* is the main contaminant in the first few days postpartum, while *C. pyogenes* is the most important bacteria in the later postpartum period, associated with animals with endometritis (WILLIAMS et al., 2007). This bacteria is rarely isolated alone, but is associated with other microorganisms, mainly the gram-negative anaerobic bacteria *Bacteroides spp.* and *Fusobacterium necrophorum* (DOHMEN et al. 1995).

Normally, infections start with gram-negative microorganisms, subsequently making the environment favorable for gram-positive ones.

1. Pathogenic bacteria:	*A. pyogenes*
	P. melaninogenicus
	E. coli
	F. necrophorum
	F. nucleatum
	Proteus spp.

2. Potentially pathogenic bacteria:	*Bacillus licheniformis* *Enterococcus faecalis* *Manhemia haemolytica* *Pasteurella multocida* *Staphylococcus aureus* Non-hemolytic *Streptococcus* *Haemmophilus sommus* *Streptococcus uberis*
3. Opportunistic bacteria:	*Clostridium perfringens* *Klebsiella pneumoniae* *Micrococcus spp.* *Proteus spp.* Coagulase-negative *Staphylococcus spp.* *Alpha hemolytic streptococcus* *Aspergilus spp.* *Clostridium spp.*

Table 4: Microorganisms isolated and identified from uterine infections in cows and their pathogenicity.

Adapted from WILLIAMS et al. (2005), SHELDON & DOBSON (2004) and BONDURANT (1999).

Most of these microorganisms are opportunistic, i.e. they are normal inhabitants of the urogenital tract. When the animal's immune system is weakened due to stress factors, sanitary problems and overcrowding, these microorganisms find favorable conditions for proliferation, becoming pathogenic (MURTHY et al., 1974, VERMA et al., 1997), determining the occurrence of the disease.

6. PATHOGENESIS OF ENDOMETRITIS

The bovine uterus is sterile before parturition. During pregnancy, the cervix and mucous plug act as a physical barrier against intrauterine invasion by microorganisms (SHELDON & DOBSON, 2004). It is important to differentiate between physiological bacterial contamination of the uterine lumen postpartum and the persistence of pathogenic bacteria with the establishment of uterine disease (SHELDON, 2004). According to FOLDI et al. (2008), *Streptococcus spp., Staphylococcus spp.* and *Bacillus spp.* are isolated from the uterus of cows with normal uterine involution, while *C. pyogenes, E. coli* and gram-negative anaerobic bacteria are found in the uterus of cows affected by uterine disease. These microorganisms, besides being the most important pathogens in uterine infections, are also responsible for infertility, damage to the endometrium and alterations in ovarian function.

Bacterial contamination does not always lead to disease (SHELDON et al., 2007), as the immune system is usually able to fight off the infection. The percentage of animals with bacteria in utero decreases as the postpartum period progresses (WILLIAMS et al., 2005).

For infection to occur, pathogenic bacteria must adhere to the mucosa, colonize it, penetrate the epithelium and/or release bacterial toxins. The development of uterine disease also depends on the cow's immunity, as well as the bacterial species and load. The number of pathogenic bacteria in the uterus of postpartum cows can be large enough to overcome the defense mechanisms of the uterus and cause infection (SHELDON et al., 2006; SHELDON & DOBSON, 2004).

7. PREVENTION OF ENDOMETRITIS

To minimize the damage caused by endometritis on dairy farms, the best way is to prevent it is through nutrition and cow management during the transition period. Cows with a low body condition score at calving are more predisposed to dystocia, metabolic disorders, retained placenta and later development of uterine infections (HOEDEMAKER et al., 2009; ZABORSKI et al., 2009). Similarly, overfed cows with a body condition score of 4 on a 5-point scale have a higher risk of developing postpartum endometritis (URTON et al., 2005; BACHA & RAGASA, 2010).

BELL & ROBERTS (2007) showed the importance of monitoring body condition during lactation and in the transition period, in which the body condition score should be equal to 3.5. HUZZEY et al., (2007) showed that one of the most effective ways to avoid uterine infections in the postpartum period is to ensure a high dry matter intake during the transition period.

During inflammatory processes, free radicals are released which reduce the action and lifespan of antibodies, damaging the immune system. Micro minerals such as copper, selenium, zinc and manganese are directly linked to animal immunity and are responsible for reducing the action of these free radicals (BORGES & PASCHOAL, 2012). Calcium, phosphorus, sodium and potassium, among other macro minerals, also play a role in the immune function of animals, since levels below the required level lead to a drastic decrease in the action of macrophages and natural killer cells, as well as the deregulation of sodium and potassium pumps in cells, causing damage to the cell membrane (GONZALES et al., 2000).

Another very important factor is hygiene in the maternity pen, as it influences the incidence of postpartum uterine infections (LEWIS, 1997; OPSOMER & KRUIF, 2009). PALMER (2005) and BELL & ROBERTS (2007) reported that in a dirty environment, there is great bacterial multiplication, increasing the chance of contamination both pre-partum and post-partum.

Genetic factors can also predispose to the development of endometritis in the event of obstetric complications (JOOSTEN et al., 1991; ZABORSKI et al., 2009). For this reason, genetic selection is important in an attempt to reduce the occurrence of dystocia, such as the use of semen from bulls approved for calving ease in the artificial insemination of heifers (CARNIER et al., 2000; POTTER al et., 2010).

Knowing that retained placenta is a significant risk factor for uterine infection and, as its cause is multifactorial, it is difficult to come up with a single way of preventing this from occurring (LEBLANC, 2008). Aspects that decrease immune function at the end of pregnancy and in the recent postpartum period predispose cows to secondary retention (ABDELHAMEED et al., 2009), as does vitamin E and D deficiency (ALSIC et al., 2008). According to SATTAR et al. (2007) and COOK & GREEN (2007), a prepartum diet containing 0.1 - 0.5mg/day of selenium, 100g/day of calcium and 2000 IU of vitamin E is an effective way of reducing the incidence of retained placenta. This is because vitamin E is responsible for the activity of the enzyme glutathione peroxidase in the placenta and its deficiency results in decreased prostaglandin synthesis, affecting the contraction activities of the myometrium (GAJEWSKI et al., 1999; ABDELHAMEED et al., 2009).

For BLOOD & RADOSTITIS (2000), the control of infectious diseases such as Bovine Brucellosis, Campylobacteriosis, Infectious Bovine Rhinotracheitis (IBR), Bovine Viral Diarrhea (BVD) and Leptospirosis, which interfere with reproduction by increasing cases of retained placenta, can contribute to reducing the incidence of uterine infections.

Finally, knowing the risks of endometritis in animals with dystocia that have undergone obstetric maneuvers including caesarean sections and fetotomies, immediate gynecological examination is recommended to look for injuries to the soft fetal tract and to perform uterine lavage for cleansing, in addition to paying attention to the subsequent occurrence of retained fetal membranes (GRUNERT et al., 2005).

8. CLASSIFICATION OF ENDOMETRITIS

Endometritis and metritis must be differentiated because they are mistakenly used as synonyms in the diagnosis of uterine infections after childbirth.

Endometritis is inflammation of the endometrium and metritis refers to inflammation of all uterine layers (CAMPOS et al., 2011), involving the endometrium, myometrium and glandular tissues, and is usually accompanied by a clinical picture of endotoxemia (RADOSTITS et al., 2002).

Endometritis, also known as genital catarrh, is associated with delayed uterine involution (GRUNERT et al., 2005). It is characterized by inflammation of the endometrium with varying degrees of damage to the uterine epithelium (RADOSTITIS, 2002) and can persist for a long period, characterizing chronic endometritis, leading to fibrosis of the uterine lumen, compromising the animal's reproductive life (SANTOS, 2009).

The definition and characterization of the various manifestations of uterine disease vary between research groups. According to the German Veterinary School, Hannover, the classification of endometritis is based on the presence of uterine discharge associated with cervical involvement, and is divided into 4 groups as shown in Table 3.

Classification of genital catarrh	**Characterization and manifestation**	**Characteristics of uterine discharge**
1st degree genital catarrh (CGI)	Cervicitis and chronic post-puerperal endometritis	Sero-mucous

2nd degree genital catarrh (CGII)	Cervicitis and mucopurulent post-puerperal endometritis	Mucous with streaks of pus
3rd degree genital catarrh (CGIII)	Cervicitis and chronic purulent post-puerperal endometritis.	Purulent
4th degree genital catarrh (CGIV)	Closed pyometra	Purulent
		(when cervix open)

Table 5: Classification of endometritis.
Source: GRUNERT et al., 2005.

The clinical signs manifested by cows affected by endometritis allow us to characterize the four clinical forms, which do not represent different diseases, but only a variation in their severity. According to GRUNERT et al. (2005), for the diagnosis, prognosis and treatment of uterine infections in cows, it is very important to consider the gynecological clinical picture as follows.

1st degree genital catarrh is characterized as an inflammatory process that affects the mucosa of the female genital tract, resulting in reduced reproductive performance in the absence of signs of clinical endometritis. Cows with CGI have normal cyclicity and mucous vaginal flow with barely perceptible turbidity, known as dirty mucus. Rectal palpation shows no obvious alterations, but vaginoscopy shows a slightly open cervix with hyperemic mucosa, greater moisture in the vaginal mucosa, even in the progesterone phase of the estrous cycle and prolapse of the first cervical ring, which is the sign used to diagnose subclinical endometritis.

Second-degree genital catarrh is characterized by mucopurulent vaginal discharge, which may or may not be associated with cervicitis or vaginitis. Estrus in sick cows is regular, and there is always a return after several inseminations (Repeat breeder). The corpus luteum may persist due to damage to the endometrium, making it impossible or deficient to produce PGF2a and consequently absent luteolysis. Rectal palpation shows a flaccid uterus with no contractility. Vaginoscopy shows mucopurulent flow, increased vaginal moisture and hyperemic mucosa, characterizing cervicitis.

3rd degree genital catarrh is a generalized inflammatory process of the endometrium and cervix, the clinical manifestations are more severe, compromising the regularity of the estrus cycles, with a period of acyclia, with purulent genital flow. Rectal palpation shows an increase in the consistency of the uterus with thicker walls as a result of inflammation, and an increase in the volume of the organ can be detected due to the accumulation of purulent material. Palpation of the ovaries shows a persistent corpus luteum. Indirect inspection of the vagina using a vaginoscope shows increased humidity, purulent discharge and cervicitis.

The inflammatory process characterized by 4th degree genital catarrh presents as an accumulation of pus in the uterine cavity, called pyometra. Pyometra can also result from the death of the embryo or fetus with subsequent infection by *C. pyogenes.* In this degree of endometritis, the cervical canal is closed, however, at times the cervix may open with purulent vaginal flow. In pyometra, cows don't cycle due to the presence of a persistent corpus luteum, which can lead to the thought that there is a pregnancy, as there is no PGF2a production due to the uterine contents and so there is no luteolysis and uterine contraction to evacuate the purulent material. Gynecological examination by rectal palpation reveals an increase in the volume of one or both uterine horns and increased tension in the wall of the organ. In cases of closed pyometra, vaginoscopic examination does not reveal any significant information, as the mucosa is dry and pale due to the influence of progesterone. On ultrasound, pyometra presents as an accumulation of contents with mixed echogenicity in the uterine lumen, distension of the uterus with a thick and swollen uterine wall. The condition is rarely accompanied by systemic disease.

Clinical endometritis affects 15-20% of cows between 4 and 6 weeks after calving, and around 30-35% of females have subclinical endometritis between 4 and 9 weeks after calving (LEBLANC, 2008).

The chronification of acute endometritis is one of the main causes of infertility or sub-infertility in cows, as it is usually not checked in the puerperium, due to poor assessment of vaginal mucus and the non-use of a speculum to check the internal mucous membranes (BLOOD & RADOSTITIS, 1991).

9. CONSEQUENCES OF ENDOMETRITIS

Among the problems caused by uterine infections, the economic damage is not limited to the cost of treating the animal. Uterine infections increase the calving interval, which means fewer calves and milk produced per year and an increase in the number of inseminations (MOSS et al., 2002; ANDRADE et al., 2005), resulting in a greater number of doses of semen spent per pregnancy. This is in addition to secondary infertility or subfertility, which leads to the early disposal of animals of reproductive age (SHELDON et al., 2007).

The presence of pathogenic bacteria in the uterus causes inflammation, histopathological lesions in the endometrium, delayed involution of the uterus and decreases the chance of embryo survival. Cows with a history of repeated oestrus usually have a uterine bacterial population composed of *E.coli, Staphylococcus aureus* and *C. pyogenes,* making the uterus an unviable environment for sperm survival due to the altered pH (MURTHY et al., 1974).

In addition, bacterial metabolites and the associated inflammation suppress the secretion of LH from the pituitary gland, disrupting ovarian follicular growth in the postpartum period, which interrupts ovulation in cows. Thus, uterine disease is associated with lower pregnancy rates, increased calving to first service intervals and increased culling rates due to reproductive problems (LEBLANC et al., 2002; SHELDON et al., 2006).

Long luteal phases can also occur, associated with greater production of PGE2 by endometrial cells than PGF2a (HERATH et al., 2009) and altered ovarian cycles, such as prolonged anestrus, prolonged luteal function and ovarian cysts (MATEUS et al., 2002; BALOGH et al., 2008). Therefore, bacterial infections, more specifically bacterial components such as lipopolysaccharide (LPS), not only alter uterine function, but also ovarian function and the control centers in the hypothalamus and pituitary gland (SHELDON et al., 2009). Cows with uterine disease that ovulate have low concentrations of peripheral plasma progesterone, which can further reduce the possibility of conception associated with endometritis (SHELDON et al., 2009).

Cows affected by retained placenta and/or acute endometritis are predisposed to other diseases such as ketosis, abomasal displacement and ovarian cysts. Studies based on American and European data have shown that cows with retained placenta are 2.2 times more likely to have left abomasal displacement and 6.0 times more likely to develop endometritis (OPSOMER, 2009).

10. DIAGNOSIS

According to the table below, the diagnosis of endometritis should be based on a history of recent calving (eutocic or dystocic), signs of anorexia, weight loss and a drop in milk production and uterine discharge, as well as a general clinical examination and a gynecological examination of the cow.

1. Anamnesis of the cow	- Animal identification - Recent childbirth - Information about the immediate postpartum period - Milk production - Risk factors
2. General clinical examination	- Heart and respiratory rates - Rumen frequency - Temperature - Coloration of mucous membranes - Concomitant diseases
3. Gynecological examination:	- External examination - Rectal palpation - Ultrasound - Vaginoscopy
4. Complementary exams:	- Cytology - Uterine biopsy - Culture and antibiogram

Table 6: Examination of the cow's genital system.

According to GRUNERT et al. (2005), it is essential that the veterinarian has knowledge of semiology, so that during the clinical examination the evolution of the puerperium can be evaluated, allowing to establish if it occurs within physiological standards or if it presents pathological alterations.

It is recommended that calved animals undergo a gynecological examination between the 25th and 30th day after calving. This allows time for cows with genital catarrh to be diagnosed and treated immediately, so that at the end of the puerperium, they are in a position to be inseminated, avoiding an increase in the service period due to uterine inflammation of infectious origin (PAISLEY et al., 1984).

10.1 ANAMNESIS AND GENERAL CLINICAL EXAMINATION

Before carrying out the gynecological examination itself, it is necessary to take a patient history, which should include information on the cow's identification, breed, age, date, progress and outcome of the previous pregnancy; elimination or not of the placenta after calving; progress of the puerperium; behavior and duration of the estrous cycle; insemination or natural mating; any previous treatment; stage of lactation and daily milk production (DIRKSEN et al, 1993).

Once the anamnesis has been completed, a general clinical examination is carried out on the animal while it is at rest and on the move. When assessing the animal's general condition, habits and attitudes are taken into account, since diseases affecting the female genital tract can alter the animal's constitution, temperament, character and nutritional conditions.

10.2 EXTERNAL EXAMINATION

This includes inspecting the perineal region for traces of mucus or crusts of secretion that indicate oestrus or the presence of genital catarrh. The lips of the vulva should be inspected for position, size and degree of closure, and the hairs on the ventral commissure should be checked for dryness, dampness or adhesions of mucus and/or feces. Inspection of the vulva is completed by assessing the mucosa of the vulvo-vestibular region (DIRKSEN et al., 1993).

10.3 INTERNAL EXAMINATION

10.3.1 RECTAL PALPATION

Through transrectal palpation, the size, symmetry, contour, consistency and contractility of the uterine horns can be assessed, but as it is a subjective method, it does not make it possible to distinguish between normal and abnormal uterine involution (LEWIS, 1997), and it is not very sensitive or specific for diagnosing endometritis (YOUNGQUIST & SHORE, 1997). Tables 7, 8 and 9 show the parameters that should be assessed during the rectal palpation examination.

Uterus size	
U I	Uterus held in the hand and uterine horns as thick as a finger
U II	Uterus held in the hand and uterine horns as thick as two fingers
U III	Uterus collected in the hand and uterine horns with a thickness of three fingers
U IV	Uterus delimited with the hand and curvature greater than the size of the human forearm
U V	Uterus almost delimited by the hand and curvature greater than the human forearm
U VI	Uterus not delimited with hand

Table 7: Uterus size.

Symmetry of the uterine horns	
S	Uterine horns of the same size (Symmetrical)
AS	Uterine horns of different sizes (asymmetrical)
AS++	Right horn much larger than left horn
+ AS	Left horn larger than right horn

Table 8: Symmetry of the uterine horns.

Consistency and contractility of the uterus	
C I	Uterus not very contracted
C II	Moderate contractility
C III	Strong contractility

Table 9: Consistency and contractility of the uterus.

10.3.2 ULTRASOUND

Ultrasound is another method used to diagnose endometritis, as it makes it possible to verify the presence and characteristics of the contents inside the uterus, the appearance of the endometrium, as well as offering the advantage of an immediate diagnosis. To carry out this examination, it is recommended to use a rectal or sectoral transducer with a frequency of 5 to 10MHz (DIRKSEN et al., 1993). However, the need for practice on the part of the veterinarian and the high cost of the devices have limited their use (MORTIMER et al., 1997).

Ultrasound makes it possible to differentiate between normal and delayed uterine involution (SIMOES et al., 2004). In the process of normal uterine involution, a small amount of fluid is observed inside the uterus, which is not always perceptible on rectal palpation, in the period between the final phase of loquio elimination and the end of the uterine involution process. On the ultrasound image, this fluid is characterized by a small anechoic area inside the uterus. In the presence of infectious processes, different amounts of content are observed in the horns containing purulent material in suspension, which is visualized as hyperechoic particles in motion. In the presence of inflammatory processes, the uterine wall may be thickened (SIMOES et al., 2004).

The greater the amount of content present in the uterine lumen, the greater the degree of bacterial contamination and the severity of puerperal infections (KASIMANICKAM et al., 2004; BARLUND et al., 2008).

10.3.3 VAGINOSCOPY

The next stage of the gynecological examination involves indirect inspection of the vagina and cervix, using Gotze's tubular vaginal speculum or Polansky's flambé speculum, with prior dry cleaning of the vulva, anus and their surroundings (DIRKSEN et al., 1993).

With the vaginal insertion of the vaginal speculum, the shape and degree of opening of the cervix, the color and moisture of the vaginal mucosa are assessed, as shown in tables 10, 11, 12 and 13.

Cervix shape	
C	Vaginal projection of the cervix is contracted and conical in shape
R	Vaginal projection of the cervix relatively loose and rosette-shaped
F	Widening and loosening of the vaginal projection of the cervix, which may be lobed and pendulous.

Table 10: Shape of the vaginal projection of the cervix.

Degree of opening of the cervical canal	
0	The orifice of the cervical canal is closed
1	Cervical hole for a straw (approximately 3mm in diameter)
2	Pervasive cervical orifice for a pencil
	(approximately 7mm in diameter)
3	Pervious cervical orifice for a finger (approximately 15mm in diameter)
4	Cervical orifice for two fingers (30mm diameter)
5	Pervious cervical orifice for three fingers (45mm diameter)

Table 11: Degrees of opening and characteristics of the vaginal projection orifice of the cervix.

Color of the mucosa	
A	Faded pink/pale pink coloration
B	Pink color without signs of irritation or inflammation
C	Reddish-pink color (hyperemic)
D	Fornix in red
E	Intense red coloration limited to the spiral folds of the canal

Table 12: Coloration of the vaginal mucosa and cervix projection (fornix).

Degree of humidity	
I	Mucosa is dry and sticky, no secretions have accumulated
II	Less moisture, less viscous mucus
III	Moderate degree of mucosal moisture; shiny mucosa

IV	Intense moisture of the mucosa; cords of viscous mucus between the ventral and dorsal portions of the vagina
V	Accumulation of fluid in the vagina. Depending on its origin, designated by a small letter (m = mucus; s = blood; p = pus; mp = mucopurulent).

Table 13: Degrees of humidity of the vaginal mucosa and vaginal projection of the cervix.

Vaginoscopy is one of the most important diagnostic techniques and has some advantages, such as low cost, speed and ease of examination (SHELDON & DOBSON, 2004; WILLIANS et al., 2005; GAUTAM et al., 2010), as well as detecting abnormal secretion in the vagina and cervix (LEBLANC et al., 2002; REBHUN et al., 2000). The assessment of vaginal discharge is one of the most important tools for diagnosing uterine disease, as the presence of pus in the vagina is related to the presence of pathogenic bacteria in the uterus (DOHMEN et al., 1995; LEBLANC et al., 2002; WILLIAMS et al., 2005).

The appearance and smell of this discharge indicate the degree of endometrial involvement (STUDER & MORROW, 1978; SHELDON & DOBSON, 2004; WILLIANS et al., 2005). According to LEBLANC et al. (2002), clinical endometritis can be diagnosed by assessing the appearance of the uterine discharge detected by vaginoscopy.

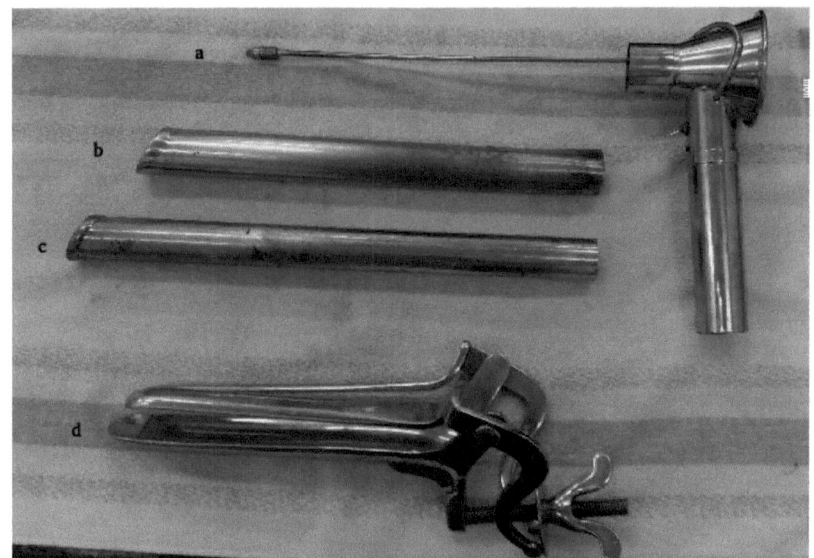

Figure 3: Equipment used in the gynecological examination of cows: A, Light source; B, Gotze small tubular speculum; C, Gotze large tubular speculum; D, Polansky speculum. **Source:** Personal archive.

10.4 COMPLEMENTARY TESTS

When clinical evaluation is not enough to detect abnormalities, laboratory tests can be carried out by collecting uterine contents and/or endometrial biopsies. Bacterial culture, histopathology and cytology are examples of complementary tests carried out to detect causes of subfertility in herds with problems of repeated oestrus without an apparent cause, frequent in cases of subclinical endometritis (AHMADI et al., 2005; BARLUND et al., 2008).

There is a strong correlation between the findings of the vaginal secretion assessment and the results of complementary tests such as culture

histopathology and uterine cytology. According to FOLDI et al. (2006), samples of uterine contents should be processed within 24 hours of collection for microbial cultures, and blood agar and MacConkey agar are the most commonly used media for growing gram-positive and gram-negative bacteria, respectively (CERMENO et al., 1997; VASCONCELOS et al., 2000). Vaginal secretions with a purulent appearance are associated with the presence of C. *pyogenes, Fusobacterium necrophorum* and *Proteus sp.* (STUDER & MORROW, 1978; WILLIANS et al., 2005), and secretions with a fetid odor are associated with the presence of *C. pyogenes, E.coli* and *Manhemia haemolytica* (WILLIANS et al., 2005).

Uterine cytology samples can be obtained using swabs, biopsies or the Cytobrush gynecological brush, which is attached to a stainless rod that is inserted into the uterus. The gynecological brush is protected by a sanitary shirt to avoid contamination during passage (KASIMANICKAM et al, 2004).

The uterine lavage technique consists of infusing 10 to 20 ml of sterile saline solution into the uterus, followed by massage of the uterine horns to recover the contents for subsequent laboratory analysis (GILBERT et al, 2005). Cytology is useful in diagnosing subclinical endometritis (LEBLANC et al., 2002), since subclinical endometritis is defined by the presence of more than 18% neutrophils (PMN) in uterine cytology samples taken between 21 and 33 days postpartum or more than 10% PMN between 34 and 47 days postpartum (SHELDON et al, 2006).

Uterine biopsy allows the samples to be evaluated histopathologically and biochemically and is therefore the most representative technique. The interpretation of biopsy results must take into account the phase of the estrous cycle the animal is in, as neutrophils can be seen in healthy animals in the period close to oestrus. But in general, the presence of inflammatory cells during the luteal phase is considered pathological (STUDER &MORROW, 1978).

However, these complementary test methods are not widely used in the field because they are relatively expensive and do not provide results in real time, making them difficult to interpret.

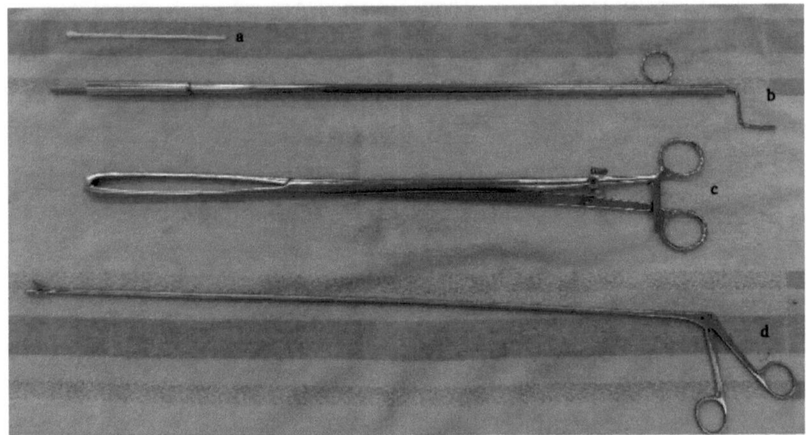

Figure 4: Instruments used to carry out examinations complementary on the cow: A, sterile swab; B, instrument for cervical swab; C, Albrechtsen cervical clamp; D, instrument for uterine biopsy. **Source:** Personal archive.

11. PROGNOSIS

The prognosis depends on the cause and duration of the condition. The more catarrhal and the earlier the diagnosis and treatment, the greater and better the prospects for restoring the cow's fertility. Sometimes, endometritis is cured spontaneously in females that are cycling due to the elimination of pathogens and the regeneration of the endometrial region.

Infections caused by *C. pyogenes* have an unfavorable prognosis, as they persist even after intensive treatment. Also unfavorable are cases of prolonged inflammation or repeated treatments with abrasive products that lead to the endometrium being replaced by connective tissue (BORALLI et al., 2012). The presence of ovarian structures in the ovary ipsilateral to the previous pregnancy is evidence of a good prognosis (BONNETT & MARTIN, 1995).

In cases of 1st degree genital catarrh, the prognosis is good and in some animals spontaneous healing can occur with normal estrus. For 2nd degree genital catarrh, the prognosis is poor, with a 35-50% cure rate with routine treatments (GUIDO, 2007). For 3rd and 4th degree genital catarrh, the prognosis is guarded to unfavorable for reproductive function (GRUNERT et al., 2005), with a 25% cure rate using routine treatments (GUIDO, 2007).

12. TREATMENT

The need to detect and treat animals with endometritis efficiently and as quickly as possible is very important in order to avoid effects on the animals' reproductive efficiency. The accuracy and time elapsed from the onset of endometritis to the diagnosis of the disease are essential for deciding on the management and treatment of the animal (AZAWI, 2008).

When the first clinical signs go unnoticed, the disease detected in its most progressive form can be more difficult to treat (OPSOMER, 2009). For this reason, dairy farms need to adopt monitoring programs to prevent, detect and treat uterine diseases early (SMITH & RISCO, 2005).

The prevention of uterine diseases is based on knowledge of the risk factors and mechanisms of action, involving the immune and inflammatory responses and the endocrine regulation of the uterine environment (SHELDON & DOBSON, 2004).

The general principle of treating endometritis is to eliminate or reduce as much as possible the infectious agents present in the uterus, not to cause damage to the endometrium, to stimulate the uterine repair and defense mechanisms in order to fight the infection and reverse the effect of the inflammation that causes a decrease in fertility and not to leave undesirable residues of the drugs used in milk for human consumption (GRUNERT et al., 2005; LEBLANC, 2008).

The therapeutic treatment of endometritis includes the use of antimicrobials systemically and/or through uterine infusions (RODRIGUES et al., 2008), and there may be a combination of drugs (hormonal and antimicrobial treatments) and the application of stimulants to the uterus to increase its contractility and eliminate its contents (GRUNERT et al., 2005). The success of the treatment depends on the physiological state of the female, the amount of uterine content, the susceptibility of the pathogens to the drugs and the concentration of these drugs in the uterus (BONDURANT, 1999; LEBLANC et al., 2002; AZAWI, 2008).

According to FERNANDES et al., 2012, the association of PGF2a analogues with antibiotics improves the reproductive performance of treated animals when compared to untreated animals. The improvement in uterine health and the earlier return to reproductive activity after calving is reflected in the shorter interval from calving to artificial insemination.

In some cases involving systemic involvement, the use of non-steroidal anti-inflammatory drugs and supportive therapy with intravenous or oral fluid therapy is indicated.

12.1 HORMONE TREATMENT

The use of hormones aims to increase uterine tone, favoring the drainage of purulent catarrhal secretions accumulated in the cavity of the genital tract and, to this end, estrogens, oxytocin and prostaglandins and their analogues are used.

Hormones	Dose	Comments
Estrogens:		
Estradiol benzoate (1mg/ml)	2-5ml IM	Risk of follicular cyst formation
Estradiol cypionate (2mg/ml)	1.5-5ml IM	Risk of follicular cyst formation
Gonadotropin Releasing Factor:		
GnRH	Depends on the drug used	Stimulation of follicular growth and maturation
Luteolithic factors:		

Coprostenol (265mg/ml)	2ml IM	Uterotonics
Dinoprost (6.71mg/ml)	5ml SC	Uterotonics
Uterine contractility stimulating factor:		
Oxytocin (10UI/ml)	1-5ml IM	Effective up to 12 hours after delivery

Table 14: Main hormones used to treat endometritis in cows. Adapted from GRUNERT et al., (2005).

Estrogens favor the elimination of secundins when administered in higher doses than usual and immediately after calving. However, it should be noted that the use of estrogens can lead to the occurrence of follicular cysts in cows (GRUNERT et al., 2005). Estradiol cypionate is responsible for increasing blood flow and contraction in the uterus (ANDRADE, 2002; RISCO & HERNANDES, 2003). Oxytocin is also used therapeutically, however, it should be noted that this hormone is only active in the immediate period after childbirth (GRUNERT et al., 2005).

In the presence of a corpus luteum in the ovary, as in pyometra, prostaglandin (PGF2a) should be used in treatment with the aim of promoting luteolysis, inducing oestrus, naturally increasing the blood concentration of oestrogen and regulating local immune function, resulting in an increase in the uterus' ability to fight infection (LEWIS, 1997; SHELDON, 2007). The mechanisms by which prostaglandin can improve postpartum uterine health are controversial, but aiding in the expulsion of contaminated contents and increasing uterine immunity are benefits of this drug when administered postpartum to cows with uterine infection (LEWIS, 2004; KASIMANICKAM et al., 2005; FERNANDES & FIGUEIREDO, 2007).

Hormone therapy should be combined with intravenous infusion of calcium borogluconate solution in order to stimulate uterine tone (GRUNERT et al., 2005).

12.2 ANTISEPTIC TREATMENT

The main indications for the use of antiseptic substances in the treatment of endometritis are: reducing the intensity of infection and the size of the uterus, inactivating microorganisms and increasing the tone of the myometrium due to the local irritation caused, as well as reducing the viscosity of genital phlegm, making it more fluid and favoring its elimination.

This irritating action of antiseptic solutions on the endometrium causes significant leukocytosis, equivalent to that which occurs during estrus, thus increasing the cellular defense of the tissues involved. Among the antiseptic substances routinely used in treatment are iodine derivatives, chlorhexidine and DMSO (Dimethyl Sulfoxide), applied intrauterine via the cervix using a catheter (GRUNERT et al., 2005).

Antiseptic substances and preparation of solutions	Dose
Acridine and derivatives:	
Rivanol 0.1 to 0.2%	50-150 ml
Chlorinated:	
Chlorhexidine 2-3%	50-150 ml
Anti-inflammatory/ analgesic permeability modifier:	
Dimethylsulfoxide (DMSO 5%)	30-60 ml
Halogens:	
Iodo-povidone 2-3%	50-150 ml
Lugol's solution	50-1500 ml
Oxidizing agents:	
Potassium permanganate 0.1%	50-150 ml

Table 15: Recommended antiseptic substances for the intrauterine treatment of endometritis in cows.
Adapted from GRUNERT et al. (2005).

12.3 TREATMENT WITH ANTIBIOTICS

The route of administration influences the effectiveness of treatments, as does the antibiotic used. The use of antibiotics in intrauterine or systemic treatment of genital catarrh has been widely used. The results are significantly better when the bacterial agent responsible for the infection is first isolated and identified (GRUNERT et al., 2005).

According to GRUNERT et al. (2005), intrauterine antibiotics should be dissolved in 50 to 150 ml of aqueous solution depending on the size of the uterus, with 2/3 of the volume being applied inside the uterus and 1/3 in the cervical canal.

These antibiotics are absorbed from the uterus and establish blood and milk levels, causing concern about residues in milk and disposal. Certain antibiotics can interfere with the function of phagocytic cells, be inactivated by betalactamase-producing bacteria, irritate the endometrium or may not work in the relative anaerobic state that exists in the uterus (REBHUN et al., 2000).

Antibiotic	Intrauterine infusion	Injectable with systemic action
Penicillins:	2-4 million IU	
Benzylpenicillin or Penicillin G	1-2g	20 to 50,000 IU/Kg BW
Ampicillin	5-6g	10mg/Kg BW 6g

Tetracyclines: Oxytetracycline Tetracycline hydrochloride	3-5g 1-2g	11mg/Kg BW 11mg/Kg BW
Aminoglycosphides: Gentamicin	ig	6.6mg/Kg BW IM
Neomycin Amikacin	1-2g 2g	- 2g

Table 16: Main antibiotics recommended for the intrauterine or systemic treatment of genital tract infections in cows.
Adapted from GRUNERT et al. (2005).

Microorganisms that infect the uterus of cows are generally susceptible to penicillin, but during the first month after calving, contaminating microorganisms can produce penicillanases. Therefore, some authors cite that penicillin is probably not effective during the early postpartum period. However, it is effective for treatment when administered systemically (SMITH et al., 2006).

The antibiotics used systemically to treat endometritis are long-acting oxytetracyclines for animals with low milk production due to the need to discard the milk and cephalosporins for animals with high milk production, as they do not require discarding the milk (DRILLICH et al., 2006). The doses are 20mg/kg IM or subcutaneously for oxytetracycline LA and 1 to 2 mg/kg IM for ceftiofur.

With regard to the intrauterine treatment of endometritis, the administration of cephapirin and first-generation cephalosporins is capable of improving reproductive performance in dairy cows with risk factors for uterine disease (BORALLI et al., 2012). The most widely used cephalosporin is Cefapirin, an antibiotic with great activity against Gram-positive bacteria, and the development of resistance is rare. However, there are some disadvantages to intrauterine treatment, such as the occurrence of lesions in the endometrium due to the use of irritating drugs, inadequate diffusion of the drug in the uterine wall and the inactivation of the drug in the presence of organic material (pus) in the uterus. According to GRUNERT et al. (2005) and JUNIOR (2011), the use of oxytetracycline by the intrauterine route is not recommended due to the possibility of causing irritation to the lumen, increasing local inflammation and the risk of damaging the infected mucosa at the time of application, opening the door to systemic circulation.

Intrauterine treatment of 1st degree genital catarrh can be carried out with non-oily penicillin diluted in saline solution 12 to 24 hours after artificial insemination, once the CGI cow is in regular oestrus. In cases of 2nd degree genital catarrh, treatment can be carried out with the use of prostaglandins 11 days after estrus, promoting the migration of macrophages to the uterus, reducing the interval between estrus. If necessary, the use of antibiotics such as oxytetracycline is recommended (GUIDO, 2007). In the case of 3rd degree genital catarrh, prostaglandin is applied to luteolize the corpus luteum and the animal will come into heat and eliminate the purulent contents. Uterine infusions with antibiotics (usually for two days) are required every estrus. The treatment should be repeated every 11 days (PGF2a + infusion), until the mucus becomes clear (GUIDO, 2007 and FERNANDES & FIGUEIREDO, 2007). In cases of closed pyometra, 3 applications of prostaglandin should first be carried out with an interval of 10 days and an intrauterine application of povidone iodine solution when the cow comes into heat. However, as it has an unfavorable prognosis for fertility, it is recommended to discard the animal with pyometra (GUIDO, 2007).

The presence of fever is the most common criterion used to verify the effectiveness of treatment, in addition to monitoring the appearance and odor of vaginal discharge (DRILLICH et al., 2006; MARTINS et al., 2010).

13. CONCLUSION

Farmers involved in dairy farming rely heavily on their herd's reproductive indices, as it is through calving that cows are able to provide milk naturally. It is therefore necessary to recognize those animals that are most likely to develop the disease so that preventive measures can be taken, since sick cows reduce the herd's reproductive and productive indices.

REFERENCES

ABDELHAMEED AR, AHMED WM, EKHNAWY KI AND KHADRAWI HH. Strategy trials for prevention of retained foetal membranes in a Friesian herd in Egypt. **Global Veterinaria**, 3: 63-68, 2009.

AHMADI, M. R., TAFTI, K. A., NAZIFI, S., & GHAISARI, H. R. The comparative evaluation of uterine mucosa cytology with endometrial histopathology in cows. **Comp Clin Path**, 90-94, 2005.

ALSIC K, DOMACINOVIC M, PAVICIC Z, BUKVIC Z, BABAN M AND ANTUNOVIC B. The relationship between diet and retained placenta in cows. **Acta Agricultura e Slovenica**, 2: 155-162, 2008.

ANDRADE, S. F. **Manual de terapeutica veterinaria**. 2 ed. Roca. 2002.

ANDRADE, J. R. A.; SILVA, N.; SILVEIRA, W.; TEIXEIRA, M. C. C. Epidemiological study of reproductive problems in cattle herds in the Goiania dairy basin. **Arquivo Brasileiro de Medicina Veterinaria e Zootecnia**. v. 57, n. 6, p.720- 725, 2005.

AZAWI, O.I. Postpartum uterine infection in cattle. **Animal Reproduction Science**, v.105, p.187-208, 2008.

BACHA B and REGACHA FG. Subclinical endometritis in Zebu x Friesian crossbred dairy cows: its risk factors, association with subclinical mastitis and effect on reproductive performance. **Tropical Animal Health and Production**, 42: 397- 403, 2009.

BALOGH, O.G. et al. The Possible Effect of Metritis on Formation of Irregular Corpus Luteum (CL) Forms in Postpartum Dairy Cows. **Biology of Reproduction**, v.78, 2008.

BARLUND, C.S.; CARRUTHERS, T.D.; WALDNER, C.L.; PALMER, C.W. A comparison of diagnostic techniques for postpartum endometritis in dairy cattle. **Theriogenology**, v.69, p.714-23, 2008.

BELL, M.J. and ROBERTS, D.J. The impact of uterine infection on a dairy cow's performance. **Theriogenology**, v.68, p.1074-1079, 2007.

BLOOD, D. C.; RADOSTITS, O. M. **Clfnica veterinaria**. 7. ed. Rio de Janeiro: Guanabara Koogan p. 1062-1066, 1991.

BONDURANT, R.H. Inflammation in the bovine female reproductive tract. **Journal of Animal Science**, v.77, p.101-110, 1999.

BONNETT, B. N. & MARTIN, S. W. Path analysis of peripartum and postpartum events, rectal palpation findings, endometrial biopsy results and reproductive performance in Holstein-Friesian dairy cows. **Preventive Veterinary Medicine**, v.21, p.279-288, 1995.

BORALLI, I.C.; ZAPPA, V. Endometritis in cattle: Literature review. **Electronic Scientific Journal of Veterinary Medicine**, year IX, n. 18, 2012.

BORGES, L. E. M. & PASCHOAL, J.J. INFLUENCE OF MICRO-MINERALS (Cu, Mn, Se and Zn) ON THE BOVINE IMMUNOLOGICAL SYSTEM, - www.fazu.br> v. 3 (2012) Accessed on: 30/06/2017.

BRUUN J, ERSBULL AR AND ALBAN L. Risk factors for metritis in Danish dairy cows. **Preventive Veterinary Medicine**, 54: 179-190, 2000.

CAMARGOS, A. S.; GIOSO, M. M.; REIS, L. S. L. S.; COSTA, I. F.; FERRAZ, M. C.; OBA, E. Occurrence of Pregnancy, Calving and Puerperium Disorders in Dairy Cows. **Electronic Scientific Journal of Veterinary Medicine**. Year XI, n. 20, 2013.

CAMPOS & CARRER. Sterility and infertility: uterine diseases, repeat breeders and embryonic death. 2007. Available at: <http://www.camposecarrer.com.br/artigos/esterilidade.doc>. Accessed on: September 20, 2012.

CAMPOS, M. D. S. M. et al. Prevention of puerperal metritis in dairy cattle from small properties in the municipality of Pombos - PE. Available at:<http://www.sigeventos.com.br/jepex/inscricao/resumos/0001/R0072-2.PDF>. Accessed on: September 14, 2012.

CARNIER, P.; ALBERA, A.; DAL ZOTO, R.; GROEN, AF.; BONA, M.; BITTANTE, G. Genetic parameters for direct and maternal calving ability over

parities in Piedmontese cattle. **Journal of Animal Science**, v.78, p.25322539,2000.
CERMENO H, COLMENARES O, GUERRERO N, BASTIDAS P, SCARAMELLI A. Postpartum bacteriological isolation in crossbred cows with normal and pathological puerperium. **Arch Lat Am Prod Anim**, v.5, supl.1, p.594596, 1997.
COOK JG and GREEN MJ. Reduced incidence of retained foetal membranes in dairy herds supplemented with iodine, selenium and cobalt. **Veterinary Record**, 121: 625-626, 2007.
CORREA, M.T. et al. Path analysis for seven postpartum disorders of Holstein cows. **Journal of Dairy Science**, v.76, p.1305-12, 1993. DETILLEUX, J., KEHRLI, M. J., STABEL, J., FREEMAN, A. & KELLEY, D. Study of immunological dysfunction in periparturient Holstein cattle selected for high and average milk production. Veterinary Immunology and Immunopathology, v.44, p.251- 267, 1995.
DOHMEN, M., LOHUIS, J., HUSZENICZA, G., NAGY, P. & GACS, M. The relationship between bacteriological and clinical findings in cows with subacute/chronic endometritis. **Theriogenology**, 43, 1379-1388, 1995.
DRILLICH, M., MAHLSTEDT, M., REICHERT, U., TENHAGEN, B.A., HEUWIESER, W. Strategies to improve the therapy of retained fetal membranes in dairy cows. **Journal Dairy Science**, v.89, p.627-635, 2006.
DROST, M., THOMAS, P. G., SEGUIN, B. & TROEDSSON, M. H. Female reproductive disorders. Large **Animal Internal Medicine**, p. 1292-1332, 2002.
FERNANDES, C.A.C.; PALHAO, M.P.; RIBEIRO, J.R.; VIANA, J.H.M.; GIOSO, M.M.; FIGUEIREDO, A.C.S.; OBA, E.; COSTA, D.S. Association between oxytetracycline and cloprostenol in the treatment of dairy cows with retained placenta. **R. bras. Ci. Vet.**, v. 19, n. 3, p. 178-182, 2012.
FERNANDES, C.A.C.; FIGUEIREDO, A.C.S. Advances in the use of prostaglandins in bovine reproduction. **Revista Brasileira de Reprodugao**

Animal, v. 31, n. 1/2, p.108-113, 2007.

FOLDI, J., KULCSAR, M., PECSI, A., HUYGHE, B., DE SA, C., LOHUIS, J. A., COX, P. AND HUSZENICZA, G. Bacterial complications of postpartum uterine involution in cattle. **Animal Reproduction Science** v.96, p.265-281, 2006.

FOLDI J, PECSI A, SZABO J, KULCSAR M, EGYED L, HUSZENICZa G. The pathogens and cause of uterine diseases. In: International Congress on Animal Reproduction, 16, B. Workshop abstracts... Budapest: ICAR, 2008.

GAJEWSKI Z, THUN R, FAUNDEZ R and BORYEZKO Z. Uterine motility in the cow during puerperium. **Reproduction in Domestic Animals**, 34: 185191, 1999.

GALVAO, K.N. et al. Effect of intrauterine infusion of ceftiofur on uterine health and fertility in dairy cows. **Journal of Dairy Science,** v.92, n.4, p. 1532-1542, 2009.

GAUTAM, G. et al. Spontaneous recovery or persistence of postpartum endometritis and risk factors for its persistence in Holstein cows. **Theriogenology**, v. 73, p. 168-179, 2010.

GUIDO, M.C. Animal reproduction. Available at:http://www.mcguido.vet.br. Accessed on: October 17, 2012.

GILBERT, R.O.; SHIN, S.T.; GUARD, C.L.; ERB, H.N.; FRAJBLAT, M. Prevalence of endometritis and its effects on reproductive performance of dairy cows. **Theriogenology,** v. 64, p. 1879-88, 2005.

GONZALES, F.H.D.; BARCELLOS, J.; PATINO, H.O.; RIBEIRO, L.A. Metabolic profile in ruminants: its use in nutrition and nutritional diseases. Porto Alegre: Grafica da UFRGS, p106. 2000.

GONZALEZ SANCHEZ P, EURIDES D, SILVA LAF, CARNEIRO E SILVA FO, FIORAVANTE MSC, SOUZA LA, OLIVEIRA BJNA. Uterine position and uterine artery caliber in the puerperium in Gir dairy cows related to metritis and anestrus. PUBVET, v.2, p.1-9, 2008.

GRUNERT, E.; BIRGEL, E.H.; VALE, W.G. Reproductive disorders in uterus-based domestic animals. **Pathology and Chemistry of Reproduction in Domestic Mammals**, Sao Paulo, SP: Varela, p. 373-464, 2005.

HAFEZ, E. S. E. **Reprodupao Animal.** 7. ed. Sao Paulo: Editora Manoele, p. 276 -277, 2004.

HAN, I.K.; KIM, I.H. Risk factors for retained placenta and the effect of retained placenta on the occurrence of postpartum diseases and subsequent reproductive performance in dairy cows. **Journal of Veterinary Science**, v.6, p.53-59, 2005.

HARRIS, T. G., BATTAGLIA, D. F., BROWN, M. E., BROWN, M. B., CARLSON, N. E., VIGUIE, C., WILLIAMS, C. & KARSCH, F. Prostaglandins mediate the endotoxin-induced suppression of pulsatile gonadotropinreleasing hormone and luteinizing hormone secretion in the ewe. **Endocrionology**, 1050-1058, 2000.

DIRKSEN G.; GRUNDER HD; STOBER, M. ROSENBERGER. Clinical Examination of Cattle. Guanabara Koogan, 418p, 1993.

HARRISON, J.H. et al. Effect of prepartum selenium treatment on uterine involutionin the dairy cow. **Journal of Dairy Science**, v.69, p.1421-1425, 1986.

HERATH, S. et al. Bacterial lipopolysaccharide induces an endocrine switch from prostaglandin F2a to prostaglandin E2 in bovine endometrium. **Endocrinology**, v.150, p.1912-1920, 2009.

HOEDEMAKER M, PRANGE D, GUNDELACH Y. Body condition change ante and postpartum, health and reproductive performance in German Holstein cows. **Reproduction in Domestic Animals**, 44: 167-173, 2009.

HORTA, A. E. M. Physiology of puerperium in cows. VIII Jornadas Internacionales de Reproduccion Animal, AERA, Santander, p. 73-84, 1995.

HUZZEY JM, VIERA DM, WEARY DM AND KEYSERLINK MAG. Prepartum behavior and dry matter intake identify dairy cows at risk for metritis.

Journal of Dairy Science, 90: 3220-3233, 2007.
JOOSTEN I, ELDIK P, ELVING L, VAN DER MEY GJW. Factors affecting occurrence of retained placenta in cattle: effect of sire on incidence. **Animal Reproduction Science**, 25: 11-22, 1991.
JUNIOR, A. P. M. Diagnostic approach and treatment of uterine infection in cows. **Revista Brasileira de Reprodugao Animal.** v. 35, n. 2, p. 293-298, 2011.
KASIMANICKAM, R. et al. Endometrial cytology and ultrasonography for the detection of subclinical endometritis in postpartum dairy cows. **Theriogenology**,v.62, p.9-23, 2004.
KASIMANICKAM, R. et al. The effect of a single administration of cephafirin or cloprostenol on the reproductive performance of dairy cows with subclinical endometrits. **Theriogenology,** v. 63, p. 818-830, 2005.
KASK K, KURYKIN J, LINDJARV R, KASK A, KINDAHL H. Assessment of early postpartum reproductive performance in two high Estonian dairy herds. **Acta Vet Scand**, v.44, p.131-143, 2003.
KIM, I.H.; KANG, H.G. Risk factors for postpartum endometritis and the effect of endometritis on reproductive performance in dairy cows in Korea. **Journal of Reproduction and Development**, v.49, p. 485-91, 2003.
KOZICKI LE. Physiological and pathological aspects of puerperium in cattle. **Arch Vet Sci.,** v.3, p.9-19, 1998.
KOZICKI LE, BOSTEDT H, FINGER KI, ARNSTADT I. Clinical findings of the reproductive tract of cows in puerperium and their relationship with progesterone. **Rev Set Cienc Agr,** v.6, p.45-49, 1984.
KONYVES, L.; SZENCI, O.; JURKOVICH, V.; TEGZES, L.; TIRIAN, A.; SOLYMOSI, N.; GYULAY, G.; BRYDL, E. Risk assessment of postpartum uterine disease and consequences of puerperal metritis for subsequent metabolic status, reproduction and milk yield in dairy cows. **Acta Veterinaria Hungarica**. v. 57, n.1, p.155-169, 2009.

LEBLANC, S.J. et al. Defining and diagnosing postpartum clinical endometritis, and its impact on reproductive performance in dairy cows. **Journal of Dairy Science**, v.85, p.2223-2236, 2002.

LEBLANC, S.J., DUFFIELD, T.F., LESLIE, K.E., BATEMAN, K.G., KEEFE, G.P., WALTON, J.S., JOHNSON, W.H. The effect of treatment of clinical endometritis on reproductive performance in dairy cows. **Journal Dairy Science**, v.85, p.2237-2249, 2002.

LEBLANC, S.J. Special Issue: Production diseases of the transition cow. Postpartum uterine diseases and dairy herd reproductive performance: A review. **Veterinary Journal**; v.176, n.1, p.102-114, 2008.

LeBLANC, S. J.; OSAWA, T.; DUBUC, J. Reproductive tract defense and disease in postpartum dairycows. **Theriogenology**. v. 76, n. 9, p. 1610-1618, 2011.

LEWIS GS. Uterine health and disorders. **Journal of Dairy Science**, 80: 984994, 1997.

LEWIS, G.S. Steroidal regulation of immune defenses. **Animal Reproduction Science**, v. 82, p. 281-294, 2004.

MALLARD, B.A. et al. Alteration in Immune Responsiveness during the Peripartum Period and Its Ramification on Dairy Cow and Calf Health. **Journal of Dairy Science,** v.81, n.2, p.585-595, 1998.

MARION, G.B., GIER, H.T. Histological and cytological changes in the bovine uterine epithelium. **Journal of Animal Science**, v. 18, p.1552-1553, 1959.

MARKUSFELD O. Periparturient traits in seven high dairy herds. Incidence rates, association with parity, and interrelationships among traits. **Journal of Dairy Science,** v.70, p. 158-166, 1987.

MARTINS, T.M. Reproductive and productive aspects of Holstein cows and endometrial gene expression of toll-like receptors and p-defensin 5 after calving. 2010. 137f. Dissertation (Masters in Veterinary Medicine) - Federal University of Minas Gerais, Veterinary School, Belo Horizonte, MG, 2010.

MATEUS, L.; COSTA, L.L.; BERNARDO, F.; SILVA, J.R. Influence of Puerperal Uterine Infection on Uterine Involution and Postpartum Ovarian Activity in Dairy Cows. **Reproduction in Domestic Animals**, v.37, n.1, p.3135, 2002.

MOSS N, LEAN LJ, REID SWJ, HODGSON DR. Risk factors for repeat breeder syndrome in New South Wales dairy cattle. **Preventive Veterinary Medicine**, 54: 91-103, 2002.

MORTIMER, R. G.; FARIN, P. W.; STEVENS, R. D. Reproductive examination of the Non-pregnant cow. In R. S. Youngquist, **Current Therapy in Large Animal Theriogenology**, p. 268-275, 1997.

MORROW, D.A. et al. Postpartum ovarian activity and uterine involution in dairy cattle. **Journal of the American Veterinary Medical Association**, v.149, p.1596 - 1609, 1966.

MURTHY, G.V.K., NANJIAH, R.D., MURTHY, B.S.K. Bacterial flora of cervical mucus in repeat breeding bovines. **Indian Veterinary Journal**, v.51, p.26468, 1974.

NOAKS, E. N. et al. Arthur's veterinary reproduction and obstetrics. Elsevier, 2001.

NOGUEIRA LAG, PINHEIRO LEL, NORTE AI. Uterine involution and return to ovarian cyclic activity in Bos taurus indicus cows. **Rev Bras Reprod Anim**, v.17, p.49-56, 1993.

OPSOMER, G. Puerperium in the modern dairy cow: state of the art. **Revista Brasileira de Reprodugao Animal,** n.6, p.140-147, 2009.

OPSOMER G & KRUIF A. Metritis and endometritis in high yielding dairy cows. **VlaamsDiergeneeskundigTijdschrift,** 78: 83-88, 2009.

PAISLEY LG, MICKELSEN WD, ANDERSON PB. Mechanisms and therapy for retained fetal membranes and uterine infection of cows. **Theriogenology**, v.25, p.353-381, 1986.

PALMER C. Postpartum metritis in cattle: a review of the condition and the treatment. **Veterinary Rounds**, 3: 1-6, 2003.

POTTER, T.J. et al. Risk factors for clinical endometritis in postpartum dairy cattle. **Theriogenology**, v.74, n.1, p.127-134, 2010.

PRESTES, N. C., ALVARENGA, F. C. L. **Obstetricia Veterinaria.** 4ed. Rio de Janeiro: Guanabara, p. 123 - 125, 2006.

QUINTELA LA, PENA AI, TABOADA MJ, ALONSO G, PORTAS BV, DIAZ C, BARRIO M, GARCIA ME, BECERRA JJ and HERRADON PG. Risk factors for low pregnancy rate in dairy cattle: a retrospective study in North West of Spain. **Archivos De Zootecnia**, 53: 69-76, 2004.

REBHUN, W.C.; GUARD, C.; RICHARDS C.M. **Diseases of Dairy Cattle.** 1ed. Sao Paulo: Editora Roca, p. 379-387, 2000.

REIST, M.; ERDIN, D.K.; VON EUW, D.; TSCHUMPERLIN, K.M.; LEUENBERGER, H.; HAMMON, H.M.; KUNZI, N.; BLUM, J.W. **American Journal of Veternary Research**, v.64, p.188-184, 2003.

RISCO, C. A. HERNANDEZ, J. Comparison of ceftiofur hydrochloride and estradiol cypionate for metritis prevention and reproductive performance in dairy cows affected with retained fetal membranes. **Theriogenology**. n 60 p. 47-58, 2003.

RODRIGUES, C.F.M.; PARRAA, B.C.; SANTOS, L.M.; PINTO, E.A.T.; LOT, R.F.E. Diagnosis and treatment of endometritis in cattle. **Revista Cientica Eletronica de Medicina Veterinaria,** year VI, n. 10, 2008.

SANTOS, A.D.F. et al. Treatment of post-puerperal bovine endometritis by intramuscular and intrauterine routes. Ciencia animal brasileira. v. 10, n. 2, p. 602-609, apr./jun. 2009. SEEGERS, H. Economics of the reproductive performance of dairy herds. XXIV **World Buiatrics Congress**, Nice, France, 2006.

SATTAR A, MIRZA RH and HUSSAIN SMI. Effect of prepartum treatment of vitamin e-selenium on postpartum reproductive and productive performance of exotic cows and their calves under subtropical conditions. **Pakistan**

Veterinary Journal, 27: 105-108, 2007.

SENGER, P.L. The Puerperium and Lactation. In: SENGER, P.L. (Ed.) **Pathways to pregnancy and parturition**. 2.ed. Washington: Current Conceptions, p.327- 335, 2003.

SHELDON, I.M. et al. Defining postpartum uterine disease in cattle. **Theriogenology**, v.65, p.1516-1530, 2006.

SHELDON, I.M. Endometritis in cattle: pathogenesis, consequences for fertility, diagnosis and therapeutic recommendations. **Partners Reprod**, v.2, p.1-5, 2007.

SHELDON, I.M. et al. Defining Postpartum Uterine Disease and the Mechanisms of Infection and Immunity in the Female Reproductive Tract in Cattle. **Biology of Reproduction**, v.81, p. 1025-1032, 2009a.

SHELDON, I.M. et al. Mechanisms of Infertility Associated with Clinical and Subclinical Endometritis in High Producing Dairy Cattle. **Reproduction of Domestic Animals**, v.44, n.3, p.1-9, 2009b.

SHELDON, I.M. & DOBSON, H. Postpartum uterine health in cattle. **Animal Reproduction Science** 82-83 p. 295-306, 2004.

SIMOES P, FONTES P, ALMEIDA JC. Diagnosis of pregnancy and uterine pathologies by ultrasound in ruminants, horses and pigs. Online version. Vila Real: SDE-UTAD, 2004. 71p. (Serie didactica. Ciencias aplicadas, n.258).

SINGH, J., MURRAY, R. D., MSHELIA, G. & WOLDEHIWET, Z. The immune status of the bovine uterus during the peripartum period. **The Veterinary Journal**, v.175, p.301-309, 2008.

SMITH BI and RISCO CA. Predisposing factors and potential causes of postpartum metritis in dairy cattle. **Compendium on Continuing Education**, 24: 74-79, 2002.

SMITH, B.I. and RISCO, C.A. Management of periparturient disorders in dairy cattle. **Vet Clin Food Anim**, v.21, p.503- 521, 2005.

SMITH, P.B. **Large Animal Internal Medicine**. 3ed. Barueri, SP: Manole, p.1308, 2006.

STRATEN, M.VAN. et al. Associations among patterns in daily body weight, body condition scoring, and reproductive performance in high-producing dairy cows. **Journal of Dairy Science**, v.92, p.4375-4385, 2008.

STUDER, E. and MORROW, D.A. Relationships of post-partum genital tract examination per rectum to endometrial biopsy and uterine culture results. **Journal of the American Veterinary Medical Association**, v.172, p.489494, 1978.

URTON G, VON KEYSERLINGK MAG and WEARY DM. Feeding behavior identifies dairy cows at risk for metritis. Journal of Veterinary Science, 88: 2843- 2849, 2005.

VASCONCELOS JLM, ESPER CR, SANTOS RM, VASCONCELOS CGC, WECHSLER FS. Detection of subfertility in dairy cows through anatomical measurements of the pelvic region and genital tract. **Arq Bras Med Vet Zootec**, v.52, p.468-474, 2000.

VERMA, H.K., JINDAL, S.D., SHARMA, D. K., PANGAONKAR, G.R., SINGH, J. Etiology and treatment of repeat breeding buffaloes. **Indian Journal of Animal Science**, v.67, n.2, p.137-38, 1997.

WATSON ED, DIEHL N K, EVANS JF. Antibody response in the bovine genital tract to intrauterine infusion of A. pyogenes. **Res Vet Sci**, v.48, p.7075, 1990.

WILLIANS, E.J.; FISHER, D.P.; PFEIFFER, D.U.; ENGLAND, G.C.W.; NOAKES, D.E.; DOBSON, H.; SHELDON, I.M. Clinical evaluation of postpartum vaginal mucus reflects uterine bacterial infection and the immune response in cattle. **Theriogenology**, v.63, p.102-117, 2005.

WILLIAMS, E., FISCHER, D., NOAKES, D., ENGALND, G., RYCROFT, A., DOBSON, H. & SHELDON, I.M. The relationship between uterine pathogen growth density and ovarian function in the postpartum dairy cow. **Theriogenology**, v.68, p.549-559, 2007.

YOUNGQUIST, R. S. & SHORE, M. D. Postpartum uterine infections. In R. S. Youngquist, **Current Therapy in Large Animal Theriogenology**, p. 335-340, 1997.

ZABORSKI D, GRZESIAK W, SZATKOWSKA I, DYBUS A, MUSZYNSKA M and JEDRZEJCZAK M. Factors affecting dystocia in cattle. **Reproduction in Domestic Animals**, 44: 540-551, 2009.

ZAIN AE, NAKAO T, RAOUF MA, MORIYOSHI M, KAWATA K, MORITSU Y Factors in the resumption of ovarian activity and uterine involution in postpartum dairy cows. **Anim Reprod Sci**, v.38, p.203-214, 1995.